COMPLETE WELLNESS

HOW TO LIVE A HEALTHY LIFESTYLE WITH A HEALTHY DIET

BENSON BRIAN

Table of contents

Introduction

Eating right is the most difficult thing for some people. Whether it's because we have limited access to resources in all areas or simply because we have too much access to unhealthy foods, there are many reasons why eating healthy is a challenge.

We can eat almost any food we like and it'll nourish our body. We will manage to pass from one moment to the next and be able to call ourselves sane. But is eating a diet of processed foods and sugary drinks healthy? We can't eat any food and be healthy. And the older we get, the more our bad habits catch up with us.

It is incredibly important to develop healthy eating habits early in life, or at least as soon as possible, to prevent future problems. You don't want to wake up one day and find that you've been suffering from a nutrient deficiency for years, leading to complications that are nearly impossible to fix. We all need to take more responsibility for what we put into our bodies because if we don't, it can become extremely dangerous.of course, when we're older and can remember our mistakes, looking back is 20/20. We realize that there were things we could have done, and probably should have done, that we simply didn't do because we didn't know the ill effects or were just lazy. Simple knowledge alone is not enough to put into action the need to do something health-conscious.

 Most of the time, before we can fully understand how we are taking care of our bodies and our overall health, we need to deal with the suffering that can result from poor health decisions. Not being able to see the reality of the consequences of our actions can make us feel them.Far away and difficult to understand. We could even blow them up completely. This can be a very distressing situation, especially when you are already dealing with the side effects of a poor diet and a lack of healthy eating.

Everyone deserves the chance to become the best version of themselves, but if we don't even recognize that unhealthy eating can throw us completely off course in the present moment, then we end up saying goodbye to the best possible future.But all that can change. As you read this book, you will understand the importance of healthy eating and how food affects our bodies, and how we function.

Without understanding exactly why our bodies respond the way we do to food, it can sometimes be hard to keep track. But there are many ways you can begin to understand why eating healthy food is so important and how you can start eating healthy. Do not lose more time. We must start eating healthy today!

Chapter One

Why eat healthy?

Healthy eating is important for many reasons. Most of us are already aware of the growing obesity epidemic in North America.The United States is not even left out.There's even a term for the way many Americans eat, and it's called the SAD diet.

SAD stands for "Standard American Diet" and refers to a diet low in vegetables, high in fat and sugar, and deficient in nutrients.

Processed foods are a part of the SAD diet. These are foods that are readily available and quickly eaten and prepared, but have long-term adverse health effects.If you don't want to become obese, it's considered a good idea to avoid eating processed foods and instead focus on eating whole grains, fruits and vegetables, and meats that haven't been treated with hormones and other chemicals, which can eventually end up in your body and cause problems.

We have so many things available and the amount of money it takes to buy bad food is much less than it takes to buy good food. It seems strange that buying organic food costs more money than buying food that ultimately causes long-term health problems, but that's the rule of supply and demand.

Also, processed foods are mass-produced and make huge profits due to their convenience. For this reason, the obesity epidemic in North America is not particularly surprising in many respects. Nutrition doesn't top the list of companies trying to capitalize on people's laziness in the kitchen.

However, there are many reasons why it's important to eat healthy, and there are good reasons to avoid processed foods and the standard American diet. For example, if you don't want to be obese, be sure to check out the rest of this book to find ways to improve your diet and start a healthier lifestyle.

Another reason to eat healthily is that eating unhealthy foods and following a standard American diet high in fat and sugar can make you susceptible to disease. Diabetes can be the result of a poor diet and can often be treated with healthy eating.

Ultimately, type II diabetes is something that can be maintained and controlled with proper dietary habits and is triggered by poor eating habits. If you want to avoid such pitfalls and complications, you should do your best to be conscientious in your food choices.

Other diseases can also be caused by improper nutrition. Hypertension is common, as are other chronic diseases. Many people may be affected by osteoporosis in the future because they have not made healthy dietary choices in the past. You may have poor bone health, high blood pressure, or even heart problems. All of this can take its toll on your body and cause great stress, which can ultimately be very dangerous.

If you want to show your family that you care about them, start making decisions now that will help you stay in their life as long as possible. Poor health doesn't just affect you.It will affect the people around you too. When they see you suffer because you made bad decisions, it's quite selfish in a way. They also suffer. Do your best now to make the best decisions not only for yourself but also for your family in the long run. This book teaches you how.

Chapter Two

Understand your relationship with food

Over time, everyone begins to develop certain habits. We develop habits in all areas of our life. We develop hygiene habits, eating habits, work habits, and all kinds of habits. However, they hardly notice our habits until they do begin to affect us negatively. And even when we start to realize that our habits have little impact on us, changing them can be very difficult. Habit is something we do unknowingly. We are programmed to follow these habits, and it takes great willpower to break this cycle.

Once you begin to understand that your relationship with food has a lot to do with the habits you've created and can continue to cultivate and maintain, changing the way you think becomes much easier.

When you recognize the impact and importance of your future and make positive choices about those things, you may be more in tune with eating healthy and less inclined to make decisions that negatively impact you and your future.

To be honest, many of us seem gloomy about the future. We don't see enough reasons to change our habits because if we don't believe we have something good to look forward to, then it doesn't matter if we make excellent decisions or not. We do not see how we can truly shape our future in our best interest. Probably because we don't believe we have power over our lives.

If you can relate to that feeling, don't be alarmed. It is very common in the human experience. We are usually discouraged from taking control and using our power from a young age, and sometimes we stop believing that we have authority over our lives because other people usually tell us what to do.As a child, that makes sense. Children don't know what's best for them. But it can foster a very helpless mindset that makes it hard for us to understand that the consequences of our actions can start to shape who we are and the way we present ourselves.

Because of this, it's important to take steps to help you understand yourself and your eating habits. When did your habit start? How did you develop this habit? What are the benefits of this habit? What negative effects does this habit have on you?

Ask yourself as many of these questions as possible so you understand how the food you eat is shaping your future. Are you creating a healthy and energetic future, or are you creating a future that is bleak and potentially fraught with negative health consequences?

Please rate your sense of self-discipline below. Are you able to maintain discipline in your decisions? Or is it an area where you struggle? Discipline can be hard for anyone, and if you're having a hard time staying disciplined, you should look at different ways that you can encourage yourself to be a more disciplined person, both practically and mentally.

Only then do you have what it takes to start a journey toward healthy eating? Because like it or not, bad health options are everywhere. They are easy and addictive.

If we allow these bad decisions to influence us and do not take any steps to alter our behavior, then the consequences would be significant.

Whether you eat healthy or not. The ill effects will still take over your body, waiting to hit you when you least expect it.

Unhealthy eating is a self-destructive pattern that many of us participate in. Whether due to low self-esteem or simply dissatisfaction with our situation and lack of confidence in the future, self-destructive eating habits are dangerous. You must take a look at yourself and truly value your life and your future before healthy eating lasts.

There are many ways to do this, and if possible, you should even see a psychologist for support. Sometimes they can help us recognize biases and negative patterns in our lives that we are not yet aware of. Once you understand and accept these biases and negative patterns, it can be much easier for you to overcome them and take the necessary steps to make positive decisions.

Whether you seek the help of a qualified professional, there are many things you can do to change the way you think. As long as you understand that you are worthy of a healthy body and a positive future, you will allow yourself to take the necessary steps to get there.

But when you don't feel good, it becomes much more difficult. In general, it will help you to understand yourself, your habits, your mental obstacles, and your discipline.

We can all take steps each day to become our best selves, and healthy eating is a big step in that direction. And it is a step that we can take today.

Chapter Three

The danger of dietary trends

Dietary trends are widespread in today's society and almost all of them carry dangers. Unfortunately, most people who are desperate to make money rarely consider the long-term health effects of their products. What they care about is making money and doing something that helps them capitalize on the desperate desire of many people to lose weight quickly and easily.

There is something you have to accept if you are interested in food trends. The unfortunate fact is that there is no healthy way to lose weight quickly and easily without work, healthy eating, and exercise. Losing weight is a wonderful goal if you are overweight or out of shape and need extra mobility.

We've all had to start making better lifestyle choices at some point, and that's something we can achieve through healthy diet and exercise, rather than relying on companies that want to exploit us for money.

Some of the dietary trends are extremely dangerous and have devastating health consequences in both the short and long term expression. Many of them are based on methods that make us deprive ourselves and our bodies of essential nutrients. Sometimes it even dehydrates us.

Such food trends are extremely disgusting. They take advantage of people who want to be healthy but don't know how to do it. They prey on people, often women especially, who cave under the pressure of unrealistic beauty standards and women who are told only a certain way is worth looking at.

This is false. Whether you are weighing 100 pounds or more you have value. However, a healthy diet is one of the few ways to boost your metabolism and provide your body with the nutrients it needs to function at peak efficiency.

If you're depriving your body of the vitamins and minerals it needs to thrive, and you're relying on a diet that teaches you how to lose weight and add value when all they're after is your money, then you're on your way behind the line.The unfortunate truth about many dietary trends is that they put the body into starvation mode.

This can mess up your metabolism and cause you to gain weight even faster in the future. Don't be fooled by ads that promise you will lose weight quickly and effectively in an easy way. All this will have its price. Also, there are health trends like the hCG diet that can mess with your body and your hormones.

The irony of dietary trends is that they often make it difficult for you to lose weight in the future because you use unhealthy and difficult methods to maintain your weight. If you want to be skinny, don't trust a pill on TV to make you skinny. Eliminate unhealthy, sugary, and processed foods and replace them with healthy whole kinds of wheat and organic fruits and vegetables that don't introduce chemicals into your body that make weight loss even more difficult and ultimately wreck your body chemistry.

It may seem tempting to lose weight quickly and not have to break the negative eating habits you've developed throughout your life, but it's not healthy. You are hurting yourself and setting your body up for more health complications in the future if you are not careful in your attempt to lose weight. Be sure to do everything in your power to make the decisions that you want other people to make for themselves as well.

Do your research before you let the snake oil salesman on TV sway you. Look at these things because it pays to do the right thing and you deserve a positive future and not one complicated by the side effects of a sales pitch that is about your money and not your health.

Chapter Four

The food pyramid

Most of us have probably seen the food pyramid. Growing up, we often use the food pyramid as a guide to give us an idea of how much and what kind of food we should eat daily to maintain a healthy lifestyle.

Of course, there is always evidence that the food pyramid is flexible, but by looking at the food pyramid, you will have a general idea of what is acceptable in a healthy and nutritious diet.

While this is sometimes debatable, it's still good to eat a staple. Possibly one that you create yourself. Many people will say that eating as many grains as the food pyramid suggests is no longer considered the healthiest way to live.

In fact, with the recent outbreaks of celiac disease, many people are touting a grain-free lifestyle as the healthiest option.

Instead of relying on the food pyramid as a basic guide to healthy eating, try considering your own personal food experience and go from there. Some people are healthier with lots of grains, others are not. Use your best judgment here so that you can take steps in the right direction for your health.

The standard food pyramid recommends the following:

Rice, cereals, pasta, and bread can include up to 11 servings a day.

When it comes to vegetables and fruits, you should eat between three and five servings.

You can eat two to three servings of eggs a day, as long as you are not allergic or lactose intolerant.

When it comes to meat and beans and other things like nuts and fish or poultry, it is recommended to eat two to three servings every day.

Unsurprisingly, things like sugar, fat, and oil top the list. Because you shouldn't have too much. Rather, use them only when necessary to ensure the healthiest lifestyle possible.

Again, this only relates to the standard food pyramid. Depending on your individual needs and nutritional capabilities, you may need to modify this chart yourself. However, unless you have special requirements, this is the standard for food.

The pyramid that you can use to your greatest advantage in creating a healthier lifestyle.

Chapter Five

How food can be your medicine

Just as an unhealthy diet can make you sick, eating healthy foods can often cure you of illness and bring relief when you're suffering.

It can also serve as a preventive measure against diseases. An entire healing method called Ayurveda has been around throughout India for thousands of years.

This ancient style of healing is used to treat diseases simply by changing the diet. Food is the medicine that has kept the people of India alive for centuries. And is still applicable till date.

Many remedies are simply healthy foods with anti-inflammatory properties and the ability to nourish your body from the inside out. Everything from infections to cancer is known to be affected by a healthy diet.

And with this ancient art of healing, it's never been so obvious.Of course, many modern technologies will not look kindly on these methods because they have not been scientifically studied, but many of them have been tested for thousands of years and will continue to have an impact on the body.

Whether you believe in the ancient art of healing, the fact remains that diet can ultimately determine whether you are susceptible to disease. When you eat right, your body is stronger and can fight disease and infection much more easily than if you were malnourished on the standard American diet.

Without the proper vitamins and minerals in your body, it can be nearly impossible to combat the ill effects of a disease.Sometimes it can even cause illness. When you eat unhealthy, unprocessed foods, certain types of those foods can make you sick and also make you more susceptible to certain types of cancer.

Although cancer is still being researched and has not yet been fully understood by the scientific community to truly cure it, there are many cases where people have been able to live a long and healthy life simply by changing their lifestyle habits. Eating healthy can help alleviate the symptoms of many difficult and impossible-to-cure diseases, such as multiple sclerosis.

As long as you make sure that everything you put into your body is nutritious and provides your organs and cells with all the fuel and resources they need to keep your body strong, they will continue to do so.However, if you actively sabotage your body, it won't be able to put up the same resistance as if it were well-fed. That's why it's so important to pay attention to how you feed your body. If you don't make active and thoughtful choices about the foods you eat, you can fail in ways you'll regret for a long time.

Chapter Six

The health benefits of eating vegetables

Vegetables are one of the most overlooked foods, especially when it comes to the standard American diet. Most people don't realize the importance of providing the body with the vitamins and minerals that vegetables and greens alone can provide. Sometimes people see vegetables as a way to enhance their beauty, but when it comes to improving their health, they get a little disinterested.

However, since you are reading this book, you can be sure that you are willing and able to think about why eating vegetables is important. These are some of the best reasons to include vegetables in your daily diet.

First, the body needs fiber to get rid of excess waste. Without a way to collect and dispose of the waste, it gets stuck in the body and can contribute to weight gain and other potential complications.

So fiber is important for other reasons too as well. It can help you keep your blood cholesterol levels from rising and even prevent heart disease, or at least reduce the risk of developing it.

Folic acid is also found in vegetables, and providing your body with this substance can increase red blood cell production. This can be very important in preventing the development of anemia and can be of significant benefit, especially for women who tend to need this substance during pregnancy and menstruation.

Vegetables are also naturally rich in many vitamins such as A and C, which help fight infection and keep the body healthy. It can help you speed up the healing process and absorb iron, which is another way to fight anemia and prevent it from developing. Vitamins contain a lot of potassium and this is very useful because it prevents the body from suffering from high blood pressure.

Vegetables have been shown to reduce the risk of stroke and other heart complications. They can prevent the formation of kidney stones and prevent the breakdown of bone material. Eating vegetables is a great way to deal with type II diabetes and obesity.Plus, it can help you stay strong in the fight against cancer and cancer prevention. Perhaps one of the most

The positive aspect of eating vegetables is the fact that they are very low in fat and not high in calories.This means that you can eat as many vegetables as you want without worrying too much about gaining weight. Eating vegetables as a snack is a great way to curb cravings and focus on a healthy lifestyle.

There are so many good things about vegetables. Surprisingly, they are so rare in the standard American diet. One of the best ways to help yourself avoid processed foods that are high in fat, sugar, and salt is to start by walking around the outside of your grocery store.

Check out the fresh produce department to help you make a conscious decision to fuel your body with healthy options made from fresh vegetables, instead of skipping all the way and cheating by buying pasta and other processed foods that are low in nutrient-dense vegetables.

Eating healthy starts with choosing to fuel your body, and there are few things more nutritious than vegetables.Due to unhealthy and poor eating habits at a young age, or even self-imposed habits later in life, we often lose our taste for healthy foods, but it's easy to get back on track. Make time for vegetables in your life. It may take a little longer to prepare, but the benefits are worth it.

Chapter Seven

The health benefits of eating fruits

People who follow the standard American diet it's quite unfortunate don't eat enough fruit. The fruits they eat are mostly canned or saturated with sugar. Added sugar and fruit are definitely something that negates the health benefits that eating fruit in its natural state can provide the body.

Eating too much fruit can lead to complications, especially if you have diabetes. Fruits are rich in natural sugars, and when you squeeze them, they give you a lot of sugar without much fiber to give the body an excess.

The fiber that fruits contain makes them one of the healthiest and helps the body prevent heart disease and prevent constipation. Also, high-fiber foods like fruits and vegetables are very beneficial for weight control, as they help you feel full on fewer calories. Also, fruits are rich in many vitamins and minerals, especially citrus fruits when it comes to vitamin C.

Vitamin C is a powerhouse when it comes to helping the body heal, and when you need something to help keep your teeth and gums healthy, vitamin C-rich fruits are definitely the right thing for you.

Another thing that the fruit can help the body with is in the prevention of strokes and kidney stones. Fruits are very helpful in supporting the body and preventing and fighting conditions, such as skin diseases and heart problems. Fruit can be one of the healthiest ways to help you get a boost of energy and get rid of sugar cravings you may have while trying to cut unhealthy foods out of your diet.

As long as you don't go overboard with your fruit, like putting a ton in the blender and ending up consuming a ridiculous amount of sugar, you can enjoy a healthy snack that will satisfy your sweet tooth when you're ready to unleash the massive power of fruit.

If you are interested in the benefits that food can have on your health, both fruits and vegetables have a natural tendency to give your skin a radiant appearance and make it look much more hydrated and nourished. Fruits and vegetables are high in antioxidants, as well as vitamins and minerals that provide your body with the moisture it needs to keep your skin and appearance healthy.

It can help your hair grow smoother and healthier, and help keep your skin looking youthful. Fruit can even help you to nip acne in the bud by keeping your body free of waste products that seep through your pores and hydrating your skin. The fruit is great for hydrating the body due to its high water content and you will quickly see the benefits and this aspect.

Furthermore, the fruit is particularly good for digestion. Due to the high fiber content, it helps bind waste and helps the body get rid of things that might otherwise cause problems. That is why fruits and vegetables can also help you lose weight. Instead of allowing waste to break down and store as fat, the body eliminates it before it has a chance.Fruit is another great way to fight and prevent diseases, including cancer. Some fruits, like apples, help keep asthma at bay. Others can significantly lower cholesterol levels.

Grapes are known to be used to fight cancer as well, especially red-skinned grapes. They also help combat eye and kidney problems. If you are suffering from an infection, the berries are especially helpful. They are rich in antioxidants.

To prevent hindrance to weight loss and body problems, make sure to consume fruits and vegetables that are not treated with commercially available pesticides since they absorb these chemicals.

You can even eat dried fruits to replace sugary and unhealthy snacks and give your body a sweet snack that has plenty of nutrition to offer. Just be aware of the sugar content of dried fruit, because sometimes, when sold commercially, added sugar turns a potentially healthy treat into something that can ultimately help you gain weight.

However, if you eat fruit on a regular and healthy basis, fruit can help you lose weight. As long as you don't eat too much sugar, the fiber and water content of fruits helps your body feel full and your cells and organs stay nourished. The fiber and water content will help you eliminate the problems that contribute to obesity and you will feel a big change in your overall energy levels.

You can use this energy to exercise and push yourself harder towards a healthy lifestyle. This can be especially effective when replacing sugary junk food with healthier fruit alternatives on your journey to better health and wellness.

Chapter Eight

Meat to eat for a healthy life

Meat is considered one of the most important staples in many diet, but it may come as a surprise that some meats are healthier than others. Of course, we know the difference between red and white meat. Red meat is more commonly associated with health problems and cardiovascular problems, while white meat is considered leaner and healthier overall.

What may surprise some people is that other issues make meat unhealthy. Things like what things are fed to animals while they are still alive and what antibiotics and hormones can be injected into them to make them grow faster or produce more milk, at least with cows.

These types of hormones end up in the meat we eat and can cause problems in our bodies. Ultimately, if we are not scrupulous about the choices we make when choosing our foods, they can contribute to poor health down the road, including but not limited to cancer and hormonal changes, which can be quite debilitating.

However, if you're sure you're getting your meat from healthy sources and you're not feeding the animals too many steroids and antibiotics, then you're already ahead of the game. If not, try to research local places where you can get meat that doesn't meet dangerous industry standards.

However, despite the healthy meat options, certain meats are healthier than others. One of the healthiest meats you can eat, especially when you're trying to lose weight, is fish. Fish is lean and full of nutrients. However, you need to be careful where your fish comes from.

Some fish are farmed in unsanitary conditions, while others may come from areas that could be contaminated with mercury. For this reason, it is frowned upon for pregnant women to eat fish or shellfish.

However, finding a healthy source of fish can be very beneficial for your body. Fish is rich in omega-3 fatty acids, which support brain function and memory. In general, the body requires omega-3 fatty acids to perform well, especially in intellectual matters, since they are highly sought after.

Another good option is chicken raised in a good environment. Chicken is rich in protein. It has high protein content.They are usually raised in good conditions, or at least fed foods that don't cause the same problems for the human body as a lot of beef.

However, eating grass-fed beef from a reputable supplier can also be a good option. When you eat organic chickens, these animals are less likely to be raised with dangerous carcinogens.

Conventionally raised chickens are often given feed that increases their growth rate, which can cause serious health problems for the chickens and the people who eat them. They also receive copious amounts of antidepressants and pain relievers, sometimes even arsenic and caffeine.

Eating a lot of conventional farm-raised meat is dangerous, but if you can find a good supplier, go for it.

Turkey is another great meat, as it is high in selenium. This is good for the body, mainly because it can help eliminate free radicals and other toxic substances.

Ensure that you obtain your meat from reliable sources. Conventionally raised chicken and turkey are usually given harmful chemicals to unnaturally increase growth rates, which can ultimately contaminate human bodies with these chemicals.

Eating meat can be very beneficial for the body, as long as you don't eat meat that comes from unsafe and conventionally grown sources. The chemicals that these animals are often exposed to are extremely dangerous, both to the animals themselves and to the people who consume them. If you want to eat healthy and lose weight, it's best to avoid any chemicals that can get trapped in your body and avoid weight loss.

Even if you don't expect to lose weight, eating healthy means avoiding anything that can be harmful to the body, like hormones and chemicals that mess with our delicate systems. Fortunately, there are plenty of healthy meat sources out there, whether you want to indulge in chicken, beef, or even lamb. There are ways you can raise yourself healthy and ethically to satisfy all your cravings.

Chapter Nine

The danger of processed foods

That processed foods are dangerous is no surprise. What is surprising, however, is that they are still allowed on the shelves despite the devastating effect they have on our bodies and minds. Eating unhealthy food is not just a personal choice for some people.Due to the way the economy works, people living in poverty are sometimes forced to turn to processed foods, as they are an inexpensive and easy way to feed large families on a tight budget.

The hard part is that these foods ultimately create medical problems down the road that cost even more money than would support a large family with healthy, sustainable options. Ultimately, it seems that people with little money suffer either way.

Even if you don't have a family to support on a budget, processed foods just aren't healthy. The reason they are so addictive is their high fat and sugar content.

They are usually prepared dishes that contain pasta and an exceptional amount of sugar. Too much sugar is dangerous in general, but especially for people prone to type II diabetes. Ultimately, if you consume sugar in large amounts, you will overload your body and most likely not only become obese but also develop health problems.

Sugar can help speed up the process of diabetes because it causes insulin resistance, which ultimately makes it difficult, if not impossible, to control blood sugar levels.

If you eat these foods in excess, for example, at every meal, or at least every day, there will inevitably be negative consequences. Regular consumption of these high levels of fat and sugar can lead not only to well-known diabetes and obesity but also to heart disease and even cancer. This is extremely dangerous, and processed foods should be avoided at all costs, if possible.

Another danger of eating processed foods is that they are not only addictive but also highly artificial. Most of the ingredients in these foods do not nourish the body. Rather, they make us feel full while depriving our bodies of the essential nutrients it needs for healthy functioning.

When we eat a boring and poorly nutritious diet, we end up becoming dumb. We don't think well; we don't move well, and we don't unleash the greatest possible potential. These things are extremely harmful and can lead to a lack of coordination and even depression.

We all know that processed foods aren't as healthy as the foods we're supposed to eat regularly. Our body knows it, even though our mind doesn't. And we suffer from it. We are stressed about it.

When we indulge in unhealthy foods, our bodies know whether we're addicted or not. And whether it's an unconscious event or not, we often punish ourselves. We know we're doing something wrong. We are upset and dissatisfied with it even while processing it.

Processed foods also contain many artificial colors that are powerful carcinogens. When we eat foods that contain solid dyes, we are swallowing dyes. Do you want to eat hair dye? Not precisely. But these types of chemicals are used in food. They stay in your body and don't come out. They stain your organs from the inside. These can cause cancer and are extremely dangerous.

There are also many preservatives. Processed foods stay on the shelf for a long time. More than what is healthy. A typical bottle of milk would not last several months at a time. It would curdle and spoil. The same goes for cheese and also other foods you find on the shelves that have a long shelf life.It is important for companies to establish shelf life periods, as they can make more money by keeping their food on the shelf longer. They will do whatever it takes, whether it's healthier for the human body or not, to make sure they make as much money as possible.

Preservatives often include unhealthy and unnatural chemicals, as well as excessive amounts of salt. Both are not good for the body at all. Processed foods can lead to heart problems and high blood pressure due to the excessive salt content in these foods. High blood pressure is common among people who eat processed foods, and obesity and heart attacks are among the leading causes of death in North America.

This has absolutely everything to do with the standard American diet. The sad part is that these processed foods are extremely addictive even when you know they are unhealthy due to the chemicals and high sugar and fat content.

The body begins to crave it, and it can be almost as dangerous as a drug addiction. If you are dependent on food that is neither nutritious nor healthy can have long-term consequences for their health and development.

Processed foods also contribute to obesity because we digest them too quickly compared to foods high in healthy fiber. If we digest these foods quickly and they don't fill us up because we're not getting the fiber that makes us feel full, we're not even burning the same amount of energy that we would need to digest healthy foods.

This means we eat more and digest less, leading to faster and faster weight gain. The calories present in your body are much higher when you eat a diet of processed foods. You burn a lot more calories when you eat healthy whole foods that are high in fiber.

Unfortunately, this means that people who eat and eat processed foods will eventually gain weight, whether they like it or not. And they won't give you the same amount of energy because they're not nutritious. They are likely to make you feel tired, sluggish, and overly full because you are consuming so many more of these sugary, unhealthy foods without feeling satisfied or full.

Processed foods are not properly metabolized in our bodies. You will get fat fast. Also, they are high in fat. They are often full of hidden fats and sugars. Vegetable oil is one of the key ingredients in many of these processed foods.along with things like high fructose corn syrup, which is a big cause of weight gain.

North America is facing the worst obesity epidemic in the world because of processed foods. Hydrogenated oils are extremely harmful to health because they do not break down.They remain in your body and merge with fat cells. These oils make it much harder to burn fat. They are more difficult to remove and this type of stubborn fat can lead to obesity very quickly. The ingredients in processed foods lack most of the nutritional value humans need to reach their full potential. We need the fiber, vitamins, and minerals found in real food before we can truly thrive.

If you find it hard to avoid processed foods completely, you should eat them moderately to avoid their harmful effects.They are dangerous. They can make us feel lazy, irritable, and generally unhappy.When we deviate from a healthy diet, our mood can swing from positive to negative, and ultimately we find ourselves only eating processed foods that are too sugary, too fatty, and unhealthy. The easiest and most useful thing you can do for yourself is to provide your body with this food. Adjusting to changes in routine, like giving up processed foods, can be difficult and very frustrating.

You have to spend a lot more time in the kitchen, cooking and taking care of your health and your meals. But ultimately, eating processed foods is something that can kill you and isolate you from yourself. You're actually consuming toxins and avoiding foods that can act as antioxidants, giving you a chance to get rid of the waste you put into your body.

Processed foods are the same as junk food. You are no different. These are healthier looking junk foods. They are snacks in disguise. In order to be healthy and truly feel healthy, cutting out processed foods at all costs is the first and most effective step you can take. Be cautious of packaging that claims these foods are healthy, as they are often just snacks in disguise.

Processed foods saturate your body with fat, sugar, and salt, and deprive it of essential nutrients. Do everything you can to change your habit of relying on processed foods. Eating healthy is easy and possible if you put your mind to it.

Just think about the strategy of walking through the supermarket to get fresh produce and meat, instead of walking through the aisles filled with dangerous and tempting packaging that hides the dangers of processed foods inside.

Chapter Ten

Bring it all together with meal planning

Meal planning can be one of the most important aspects of developing a healthy lifestyle. When we cannot envision the future of our diet, it can be very easy to succumb to the temptations of unhealthy foods to which we have become addicted. Especially if our habit is to eat them instead of eating the foods that nourish us.

Meal planning is quite an undertaking. It can be a bit intimidating, especially for someone who has trouble getting organized. If you're having trouble planning meals, don't worry. There are lots of ways to start planning meals that are fun and easy, whether you struggle with creativity in the kitchen.

There are meal-planning kits you can buy. Many of them can order boxes of fresh food to cook and include recipes for you to use. This can be very useful if you are not used to cooking, which is often the case.

Especially when poor eating habits and a busy work schedule make it hard to find the time to prepare healthy, nutritious meals. Research is the first step in meal planning. If you want to be healthy, you have to evaluate your options.

Researching recipes is the best place to start. Preparing a folder full of healthy foods to try can be both fun and educational.it will teach you things you'll need to know in meals you find difficult to prepare.

Recipes can be very revealing. Especially if you are interested in making discoveries. Cooking can be a tough skill to learn, but once you get the hang of it, you will be able to make nutritious and delicious meals.

Look through cookbooks and magazines and find a collection of recipes you want to try. Start with the things that look the most delicious and nutritious, and if you're a beginner in the kitchen, you might want to pay attention to the things that seem the easiest as well.

Next, you need to organize your recipes that makes them easy to navigate. When you feel overwhelmed by a lack of organization, meal planning becomes significantly more difficult.

When you start a new habit, you want to make sure you're making everything as simple as possible. Too many changes at once can tax your system, and you should always try to make small, simple changes until they become a habit.

Make sure they are easily accessible so you can easily start preparing your food. If you use a binder, consider laminating the pages or using plastic sleeves so they won't be affected by water or other food contamination when used in the kitchen.

When organizing your recipes, it would be helpful to arrange them in the order of breakfast, lunch, dinner, and snacks. This makes it easier for you to find the right recipes once you start cooking. You can even organize your binder by day of the week and plan your meals for each day and print it in the binder that way.
There are many ways to organize your recipes. Do what intuitively makes the most sense to you. It does not force you to belong to an organization that does not work scared. Instead, make sure you're doing what works the most for you in your life.

Be sure to take regular time to search for new recipes that will inspire you to keep your creativity flowing and your cooking exciting. There are many types of recipes to try and the more you try, the more interesting it can be to embark on the journey of healthy eating!

Next, you should become familiar with software such as Excel and Microsoft Office to help you organize your meal planning. Within Excel, you'll find a variety of templates to choose from to plan your meals by day, hour, and week. This can be an extremely valuable resource!

If you don't want to use Excel, there are also apps you can download to your phone, tablet, or other device to make better use of your time and resources.

You can even go the old route and buy a notebook designed specifically for meal planning. This is an important step to make sure your meals are organized and easy to access.

A meal plan is extremely helpful when trying to embark on the journey to healthy eating. Developing good habits takes time and patience, and you'll inevitably slip somewhere along the way.

But that's not significant that you have to be down to earth! It just means you have to get back up and keep trying, because giving up is so much easier than sticking to your blueprints.

One thing that can help with meal planning is to stabilize the subject. For example, many people have specific themes like Taco Tuesday and other days associated with a specific type of food. If you think this would help get you on track, feel free to emulate this type of meal planning. This is done for a reason as it works and helps keep things simple and streamlined.

It can be very annoying to have to do a lot of planning and preparation every week or month. So if you want to keep it simple, this can be a good option. You can set a theme for all bi-weekly meals, e.g. B. Eat tacos on Tuesday one night and maybe rice and vegetables on Tuesday the next day, alternate between them.What you absolutely must do is comply with the regulations.

Without a consistent implementation, everything else becomes superfluous and difficult. One thing that can help with meal planning success is accountability. If you tell someone who knows you and cares about you that you are planning.Ask them if they would dispute to help you stick to your routine.

They can help by asking you question about how things are going and whether you're staying on track. You may need encouragement and encouragement in your efforts.Regardless of how you choose to support it, it can be very rewarding for both of you. You are a positive and supportive person. It can be a genius to know that there are people around you who want you to succeed. Just make sure you cut out toxic people who bring you down by calling attention to yourself or making you feel like you're going to have a hard time achieving your goals.

Of course, constructive feedback can be incredibly helpful, but not seeking constructive feedback can sometimes be detrimental.

Make sure you understand the difference between a toxic person masquerading as a supportive person and a supportive person who genuinely wants you to be okay. Another way to take responsibility is to take personal responsibility. Personal responsibility can be achieved through journaling and self-affirmation. It can be a good way to talk to yourself about your goals, what you do internally or out loud to help you stay focused and ask yourself if you are doing the things you want to accomplish.

If you find that it isn't, then instead of worrying about it, consider your obstacles and move on as you begin to discover them.In the end, if you try, everything will work out because you make the effort and cause positive changes in your life.

Keeping a journal is useful for many reasons. They can help you write down what you ate, when, and how much. This will give you a good idea of what you can expect from yourself. You need to address and acknowledge the things you are not satisfied with. But instead of getting mad at yourself for not being a drip right away, remember that it's a process and you have to go slowly.

Instead of completely changing your routine and planning each meal for the next month, if you've never done it before, start slowly by limiting yourself to one or two meals per week, then gradually add the rest if you're comfortable with the process.Make it something that won't shock your system. A gradual change is the most sustainable. And by keeping a journal of your experiences, you can bring up your innermost thoughts about the process and the things you might not even know were holding you back.

You'll start to see patterns in your behavior and be able to predict when and why you might be tempted to stray. Recognizing these trigger points will make it easier for you to avoid them in the future.

Meal planning can be a very fun and exciting task. Even if you're not the type to enjoy this type of organization, it can be very rewarding to think carefully about what you want to put in your body and take the necessary steps to do it. Everyone deserves the chance to become the healthiest, healthiest version of themselves, and with meal planning and a healthy dose of self-esteem, you're well on your way to a healthy eating lifestyle.

<h1 style="text-align:center">Conclusion</h1>

Starting a healthy diet can be very difficult, especially if you haven't been able to develop healthy eating habits from a young age. However, becoming a more health-conscious and proactive individual is not impossible.

Fortunately, every day that we wake up alive and breathing is a day that we can begin to improve and move forward in our lives.

Becoming the best version of ourselves can seem intimidating at first, but once you realize that every decision you make has an impact on your life, whether positive or negative, it becomes much easier to anticipate the course of your life. Bad eating habits are decisions that haunt us.

If we are not careful, we will develop health problems later in life because we are not aware of what we put into our bodies when we were young. Healthy eating and exercise are the only way to create a healthy and happy body and mind.

We get angry and restless when we are stuck in our homes all day, eating only processed foods that are high in sugar and fat, and sitting in front of the TV without exercising. The standard American diet is dangerous, and it is killing people. Don't become one of them.

Instead, make the decisions you need to truly improve yourself and become the best version of yourself you can be. Make decisions that will make your family proud and ensure your presence in their lives for years to come.

If we don't take care of ourselves, it's very selfish. There are people all around us who care deeply about who we are and the value we bring to their lives, whether we realize it or not. Everyone deserves the chance to take charge of their future and create positive change that will benefit them for years to come.

Eating healthy is just one of the many ways you can start to improve and prepare your mind and body for the future. If you want to be independent and active for as long as possible without spending thousands and thousands of dollars on medical bills and other expenses, you better start eating healthy sooner rather than later.

If not, it will inevitably affect your life, both materially and physically. By reading this book and using the information.As a result, you are now better prepared to take the first step towards a healthy lifestyle.

As you plan your meals and become more aware of why eating healthy is important, your quality of life will dramatically improve now and for years to come. All you have to do is stick with it and you'll start noticing the health benefits of healthy eating right away! All you have to do is try. You can do that!